ANAL CANCER

Essential Insights for Patients and Caregivers, as well as Steps to Treatment, Recovery, and Hope for Those Who Have Experienced Anal Cancer

CARL JUAN

Table of Contents

Introductory

Cancer of the anus, the aperture at the end of the rectum via which waste material departs the body, is known as anal cancer. The anal canal (the little tube that leads from the rectum to the exterior of the body) is a potential site of development. Anal cancer, like other types of cancer, develops when cells in the anode grow out of control.

• Squamous cell carcinoma is the most prevalent form of anal cancer and begins in the squamous cells that line the anal canal. Less prevalent kinds of anal cancer include adenocarcinoma, which originates in the glandular cells of the anus, and other rare subtypes.

Infection with certain strains of the human papillomavirus (HPV), a history of anal or genital warts, engaging in receptive anal intercourse, smoking, and having a weakened immune system are all risk factors for developing anal cancer, though the exact cause of this cancer is not always clear.

• Symptoms of anal cancer may include rectal bleeding, pain or discomfort in the anal area, changes in bowel habits, lumps or growths around the anus, and itching or discharge. A biopsy of any suspect tissue is often performed alongside a physical exam and imaging testing to arrive at a diagnosis.

In some cases, surgery, radiation therapy, and chemotherapy may all be used together to treat anal cancer. The particular course of treatment is determined by the cancer's stage, its location, and other factors unique to each patient. Anal cancer has a variable prognosis, although early diagnosis and treatment greatly enhance survival rates. If you have concerns about having or developing anal cancer, it's best to schedule an appointment with a doctor to get a proper diagnosis and tailored advice for treatment.

CHAPTER ONE
Dissection of the Anus

The anus is the final orifice of the digestive system through which waste products such as feces are ejected. It is a vital element of the digestive system and its anatomy is straightforward but crucial. Here is a rundown of the anus's most important components:

• Two muscular rings called external anal sphincters enclose the anus on either side. The contraction and relaxation of these muscles regulates the size of the anal canal. The outer sphincter is under conscious control, but the inner sphincter, which prevents the involuntary emission of excrement, is automatic and maintains a certain degree of muscle tone.

• The rectum is connected to the exterior of the body via a short tube called the anal canal. Lined with mucous membrane, it carries feces from the rectum to the exterior of the body.

• The anorectal line is the area where the rectal mucosa meets the anal canal. Columnar epithelium lines the tissue above this line, while squamous epithelium lines the area below.

- Veins known as hemorrhoidal veins form a network around the anal canal. Hemorrhoids are a painful and inconvenient disorder caused by the enlargement of these veins.

- The anal canal houses several tiny glands called anal glands or crypts. These glands secrete mucus to ease passing stool and protect the digestive tract from discomfort.

- Sensitivity to touch and pressure is enhanced by the abundance of nerve endings in the anus. This sensitivity aids in recognizing the need for bathroom breaks and aids in maintaining bowel control.

The anus is an important element of the digestive system that helps get waste out of the body. In addition, the brain and spinal cord send nerve impulses to the external and internal anal sphincters, which work together to regulate bowel motions.

The anatomy of the anus is straightforward, but it's vital for regular bowel movements and good digestion. Anal cancer, anal fissures, and hemorrhoids are just few of the medical diseases that can develop when there are problems with the anus or the structures surrounding it.

Factors and Causes

Anal cancer can have many different causes and risk factors, and it usually arises from a confluence of them. The risk of developing anal cancer is influenced by a number of factors, including:

• Having a history of infection with high-risk human papillomavirus (HPV) strains, especially HPV types 16 and 18, is a major contributor to the development of oral cancer. The anus cell changes that can result from the sexually transmitted virus HPV can cause cancer.

- Condylomata acuminate, or anal warts, are also linked to an increased risk of anal cancer because they are caused by HPV infection. Anal warts have been linked to the onset of cancer.

- Those who partake in receptive anal intercourse have a greater chance of developing anal cancer. The possibility of cancer developing as a result of HPV transmission and trauma to the anal tissue is raised.

- **Smoking:** Smoking tobacco is a known risk factor for anal cancer. It might lower the body's defenses, making it more vulnerable to cancer-causing changes like HPV infection.

• People with compromised immune systems, such as those with HIV/AIDS or those who have undergone organ transplantation, are more likely to develop anal cancer. The progression of HPV infections to cancer may be halted by maintaining a robust immune system.

• Both older adults and females have a slightly higher risk of developing anal cancer than males do.

• Women who have had cervical or vulvar cancer in the past may be at a higher risk of developing anal cancer.

• History of Anal Cancer in the Family or Individually: Having a personal or family history of anal cancer may also increase risk.

• The risk of developing anal cancer may be increased by eating a diet that is low in fiber and high in specific types of fat, according to some research.

• Anal cancer risk may be elevated in patients with Crohn's disease or ulcerative colitis, two examples of chronic inflammatory bowel diseases that cause inflammation of the anus and rectum.

A person's risk of developing anal cancer depends on many factors, and many people who share these risk factors never actually get the disease. On the other hand, even people who have none of these risk factors can get anal cancer. The risk can be reduced and the likelihood of a successful diagnosis and treatment increased with regular medical checkups, early detection, and prevention measures like the HPV vaccination. A medical professional should be consulted if you are worried about developing anal cancer.

Some people may not experience any symptoms at all, while others may experience a wide range of symptoms that can be difficult to diagnose. **It's crucial to keep an eye out for the following signs and get checked out if you notice any of them:**

• Rectal bleeding is a common sign of anaplastic adenocarcinoma. Bloody stools or blood in the toilet bowl are two possible manifestations of internal bleeding.

- Persistent pain or discomfort in the mouth, which may be described as aching, burning, or itching, is a symptom that should not be ignored.

- Alterations in Bowel Function: Alterations in bowel function, such as diarrhea, constipation, or a decrease in the size of feces, may occur.

- Some people with anal cancer develop lumps or masses in the area of their anus. These might be visible to others or detectable through introspective feeling.

• Anal cancer is one of many diseases that can cause sudden, unexplained weight loss that is unrelated to changes in diet or exercise.

• Persistent feelings of weakness and fatigue that can't be explained by other factors merit medical attention.

• A persistent feeling of fullness or pressure in the anal or rectal region has been reported by some people with anal cancer.

• Constipation, diarrhea, or other alterations to bowel regularity are possible.

- Bleeding that originates in the anal or rectal area and is not caused by hemorrhoids or other common causes is called anorectal bleeding.

- An unusual or offensive odor coming from the anal area is one symptom of anal cancer.

Having one or more of these symptoms does not necessarily indicate that you have anal cancer, and it is important to keep this in mind. However, if your symptoms persist or are otherwise concerning, it is essential that you see a doctor for an in-depth assessment and diagnosis. Anal cancer and related conditions have a better prognosis

if they are diagnosed and treated
early.

CHAPTER TWO
Staging and Diagnosis

Medical examinations and tests are used in the diagnosis and staging of anal cancer to establish the presence of cancer, its location, size, and whether or not it has spread to other parts of the body.

• The first step is typically a thorough medical history and physical examination by a qualified medical professional. They'll want to know what's bothering you, what puts you at risk, and what you know about your health in general.

• A DRE is performed when a doctor or other medical professional feels for lumps or other abnormalities in the anal or rectal area by inserting a gloved, lubricated finger into the rectum.

• To perform an anoscopy, a light- and camera-equipped flexible tube (an anoscope) is inserted into the anal canal. Using this method, abnormalities or growths can be located.

• A biopsy will be taken if any abnormal spots or lesions are discovered during the physical or anoscopy. A tissue sample is taken from the area of concern for further testing. This test is the gold standard for detecting analytic cancer.

• Imaging Tests: Imaging tests may be performed to ascertain how far the cancer has spread and how extensive it currently is. Examples of typical imaging methods are:

CT Scans (Computed Tomography)

Imaging with a magnetic resonance device (MRI)

PET scans (Positron Emission Tomography)

Endorectal ultrasound is a specialized ultrasound that can be used to evaluate lymph node involvement and tumor invasion depth.

- **Staging:** Once anal cancer is confirmed, it is staged to determine its extent and to guide treatment decisions. Tumor size (T), regional lymph node involvement (N), and the presence of distant metastasis (M) are all considered in the TNM staging system, the gold standard for anal cancer.

The primary tumor's size and spread are characterized by the primary tumor's stage, or T stage.

- N Stage: This stage indicates whether cancer has spread to nearby lymph nodes.

If the cancer has spread to other organs or tissues, it has progressed to Stage M.

- Blood tests and an evaluation of the patient's immune system, among other tests, may be performed to further evaluate the patient's overall health as needed, depending on the clinical situation.

Cancers are given a stage from 0 to 4, with higher numbers indicating more advanced disease, after the staging process is complete. A variety of factors, including the cancer's stage and the patient's general health, go into determining the best course of treatment.

An individual's diagnosis and staging results for anal cancer should be discussed with a healthcare team, which may include oncologists and surgeons, in order to create a tailored treatment plan. An early diagnosis and precise staging are crucial for optimizing treatment options and maximizing the likelihood of positive outcomes.

Alternative Treatments

Anal cancer treatment options are typically determined by the cancer's stage, the tumor's location and size, the patient's general health, and the patient's personal treatment preferences. The following methods may be used in tandem to treat anal cancer:

1. Surgery:

• Treatment options for anal cancer include: o Local Excision, in which only the tumor and a small margin of surrounding tissue are removed to eliminate the cancer in its earliest stages.

To guarantee complete removal of a large tumor, a larger margin of healthy tissue may be excised during a wide local excision.

• Abdominoperineal Resection (APR): This procedure may be required for some patients with larger or more advanced tumors. The anus, rectus, and a small section of the colon are surgically removed. Stool is permanently redirected into an abdominal bag after a colostomy is performed.

• **Radiation Therapy:** Radiation therapy is often a key component of treatment for anal cancer. High-powered X-rays are used to specifically attack cancer cells, killing them. In some cases, it may even be used instead of or in addition to surgery.

• **Chemotherapy:** Chemotherapy involves the use of drugs to kill or slow the growth of cancer cells. Since the combination of chemotherapy and radiation therapy (chemoradiation) is more effective than either treatment alone, it is commonly used to treat anal cancer.

• Targeted therapy refers to the use of drugs that attack cancer cells at a specific molecular level. They find application in the treatment of anal cancer when the disease does not respond to more conventional methods.

• The relatively new field of immunotherapy focuses on training the immune system to recognize and destroy cancer cells. In particular, clinical trials are looking into it as a possible treatment for some cases of anal cancer.

• In cases of advanced or recurrent anal cancer, participation in clinical trials may be an option for some patients. By taking part in a clinical trial, you may gain access to experimental treatments.

- Consistent care is essential alongside cancer-specific treatments. Some examples of this are relieving the patient's discomfort, minimizing the negative effects of treatment, and offering moral and emotional support.

- Palliative care focuses on improving quality of life, managing symptoms, and providing emotional support for patients with advanced or incurable forms of anal cancer. The treatment aims to make the patient more comfortable rather than to cure the cancer.

Oncologists, surgeons, radiation therapists, and other medical experts may be involved in the decision-making process. Considerations include the patient's overall health, the cancer's stage and type, and the patient's treatment goals.

Treatment options, possible side effects, and the prognosis for people with anal cancer should all be discussed with medical professionals. The prognosis and quality of life for people with anal cancer can be greatly improved with early detection and individualized treatment.

CHAPTER THREE
Managing Oral Cancer

An emotional and physical toll may accompany treatment for anal cancer. A cancer diagnosis is devastating news, and treatment can be taxing on the body.

• Create a safety net by leaning on loved ones for moral support. Communicate your thoughts and worries to those closest to you. Join a support group for cancer patients, either in person or online, where you can connect with others who have gone through similar experiences.

• Get informed about anal cancer, available treatment options, and possible negative effects. With this information in hand, you'll be able to relax and make wise choices.

• Honesty and openness in communication with your healthcare team is essential. Don't be afraid to voice your questions or concerns. They will be able to direct you and explain your treatment options.

• **Manage Symptoms:** Many individuals with anal cancer experience side effects from treatment, such as fatigue, pain, and digestive issues. Collaborate with your healthcare providers to find effective solutions for these symptoms. Possible remedies include pharmaceuticals, behavioral modifications, and alternative treatments.

• **Nutrition and Exercise:** Eating a balanced diet and staying physically active, within the limits of your health and treatment, can help you maintain strength and energy during your cancer journey. If you feel like you need to, see a nutritionist.

• Addressing the emotional and psychological effects of cancer is crucial. You may want to consult a therapist or counselor who has experience working with people who have cancer. Mindfulness, relaxation techniques, and meditation can also be helpful.

• Recognize that you may need to make changes to your routine and set goals that are attainable. Pay attention to your needs and allow yourself to chill out if you feel like it.

• It's normal to feel scared or sad sometimes, but you should try to keep a positive outlook. Pay attention to the things that make you happy and fulfilled.

- **Inform Your Family and Friends:** Keep your loved ones informed of your current health status and treatment developments. Inform them of the ways in which they can help you.

- Talking to an expert is a good idea if you need advice on legal or financial issues. It's important to be prepared for any problems that may arise during treatment and rehabilitation.

- Long-term care and follow-up should be planned for, so be sure to bring this up with your healthcare team. It's comforting to have an idea of what the coming months and years will bring.

• Don't be afraid to speak up for yourself when it comes to your medical care. Don't be afraid to raise your voice and get your questions or concerns answered.

It's important to keep in mind that everyone's experience with cancer is unique, so one person's strategy for coping may not be appropriate for another. It's normal to feel a wide range of emotions, and it's fine to reach out for support when you need it. All along the way, you'll have the support of your healthcare team, loved ones, and friends. When dealing with anal cancer, it can be helpful to take things slowly and keep a positive attitude.

Prevention

Anal cancer prevention focuses on stopping the disease before it starts. Although some risk factors, like age and genetics, can't be changed, there are things that can be done to reduce the risk:

• Infection with high-risk HPV types (16 and 18), which have been linked to anal cancer, can be avoided with the help of the HPV vaccine. It's advised for both sexes, ideally before any kind of sexual activity takes place.

• The use of condoms and dental dams, among other safe sexual practices, can greatly decrease the likelihood that one partner will transmit HPV to another. Reducing the number of sexual partners may also lower the risk.

• Quitting smoking is crucial for smokers, not just to reduce their risk of oral cancer but for their health in general. Smoking reduces immune function and raises the likelihood of developing cancer.

- The risk of developing some cancers can be lowered by eating a diet that is high in fruits, vegetables, and fiber. Saturated fats and processed foods should be avoided.

- Individuals at a higher risk, such as those with a history of anal warts or a compromised immune system, may benefit from routine screenings for precancerous changes in the anus.

- Reduce the risk of complications, such as anal cancer, by managing HPV infections with the help of your healthcare provider if you have one.

People with risk factors such as a prior diagnosis of anal cancer, a history of anal warts, or a compromised immune system should prioritize prevention measures. The risk of developing oral cancer can be reduced through preventative measures such as regular medical checkups, vaccination, and healthy lifestyle choices.

Conclusion

Rarely seen cancer that begins in the anus's soft tissues is called anal cancer. It has many potential causes, but infection with high-risk strains of the human papillomavirus (HPV) is a major one. Successful treatment of anal cancer requires early detection through observation of symptoms, prompt medical attention, and a correct diagnosis.

• Physical examinations, imaging tests, and biopsies all play a role in the diagnosis of anal cancer, while staging aids in determining the cancer's extent and directs treatment choices. Surgery, radiation therapy, chemotherapy, targeted therapy, immunotherapy, and supportive care are all possible forms of treatment. Anal cancer risk can be reduced through preventative measures like the HPV vaccine and safe sexual practices, while survivorship care focuses on monitoring and managing physical and emotional well-being after treatment has ended.

• Remember that your experience with oral cancer is unique, and your treatment options may change based on your individual situation. Having an open line of communication with medical staff, having a solid support system, and taking charge of one's physical and emotional health are all essential in dealing with anal cancer. Patients' outcomes and quality of life can be greatly enhanced through prompt diagnosis, effective treatment, and consistent follow-up care.

THE END